BREAKING FREE FROM DEPRESSION

A Book About Depression and How to Rise Above it.

Causes, Symptoms, Treatments and Stress Relieve Foods

Jesse Davidson

Copyright © 2022 Jesse Davidson All rights reserved

INTRODUCTION

Depression is similar to a "common cold" in terms of mental illnesses/disorders. It is not uncommon by any means, and it can certainly infiltrate the lives of sufferers to varying degrees. The reasons for this can be varied and complex, but from a clinical standpoint, there are clear distinctions between 'having the blues' and feeling sad, and actually experiencing moderate to clinically severe depression. Having had a Major Depressive Disorder that included treatment, I can describe depression of this type as an utter complete sensation of nothingness, often beyond feeling sad where there appears to be NOTHING left. Sadness was still present (in my experience), but most of the time there was a sense of nothingness. It was completely empty. Most people who suffer from depression lose hope and/or feel completely helpless. My battle with depression had left me with nothing, nothing, nothing.

However, whether one believes it or not, something CAN be done. There is still hope! Words can be shallow, and this should be acknowledged, but from my own experience, walking down the path of suicidal ideation, depression, denial, and so much more, a loss of hope and so on CAN actually be overcome, bit by bit over time.

Of course, there is no simple solution, and it can be extremely difficult not only for those who are experiencing depression and related issues, but also for others in their lives. What are our options? Things that come to mind for others who may be trying to help are things that should not be said, such as "just snap out of it." It does not happen in this manner. It would be wonderful, but it is, to a large extent, unrealistic. However, in my experience, will-power and a willingness to get better are absolutely essential as 'ingredients in the recipe' for progressing from total complete and utter nothingness, to stages of improvement, and ideally to a stage of sub-clinical depression (which is more-or-less not having depression any longer), but there are also other very important factors that are crucial in the recovery.

Other things (verbal comments) that are NOT particularly helpful to a person suffering from depression (and should be avoided) are: * "Oh, it's all in your head."

* "Stop wallowing in self-pity."

* "There are many people in worse shape than you."

* "You have so much to be thankful for." * "You think YOU have problems." "You should discontinue taking all of those pills."

* "Get yourself together."

* "You should get out more."

* "Oh, look, everyone gets depressed from time to time." "Don't even think about it." "You're depressing me as well."

* "I thought you were more powerful than this."

* "Have you ever tried herbal tea?"

* "We all have problems; we have to get together at some point."

Hearing these things is not helpful to someone who is depressed. A depressed person is more likely to be harsh on themselves. It's difficult to know how to assist. However, some simple things can be helpful: * "I love you." * "I care." * "I won't leave you, you are not alone." * "You are important to me." * "We will get through this together." * "I will be with you for better AND for worse."

There is no quick solution (such as snapping out of it). However, there is a lot of wonderful assistance available. I have put together this book from my experience to give hope to anyone that needs it and say you can **COME OUT** of that depressing situation. There are some excellent treatments for depression, including the importance that doctors can play in our recovery from depressive disorders.

There are many things we can do and arguably many things we should not do, although most therapists would accept many 'not to do things' as a widely accepted guide of recognized 'advice', and many 'to do' things as recommended, helpful strategies that, when put into practice, can reveal marvelous healing results one small attainable step at a time.

Is there any real hope? YES, without a doubt. It should be acknowledged that it is generally difficult work and that it may take a long time to return to what one was or to live a more sustained life than previously. How many of us have had falls in our lives? Certainly, all of us. Depression, admittedly, can be a major pit, something that appears too difficult to overcome, or even others can put us in 'the too hard basket.' Perhaps we can see ourselves as this as well, and without dismissing these thoughts, feelings, and beliefs for a moment, it is quite arguable that the consequences of such beliefs, thoughts, and general interpretation of life in a depressive state can be altered by our own disputing of such destructive patterns in our minds.

Table of Content

1. Recognizing Depression — 8
2. Symptoms of Depression — 18
3. Manifestation of Motivation — 36
4. Causes of Depression — 44
5. Treatment For Depression — 48
6. Reasons For being SAD — 54
7. Effect of Depression — 60
8. Stress Relieving Food — 62
9. Changes in Lifestyle to Combat Depression — 67

Chapter 1
Recognizing Depression

Have you ever considered the term "depression"? It implies that something is emotionally pressing down on you. It's no surprise that this causes sadness, difficulty thinking and concentrating, and feelings of despair and hopelessness. These are all symptoms of depression that cause a decrease in vitality and functional activity. Fatigue sets in quickly.

We've all been sad at some point in our lives. We were laid off. We lost someone we cared about, or a tragic event occurred in our lives. It is very "normal" to feel sad or depressed when life challenges arise; it is our brain's natural reaction to these circumstances. It demonstrates that your brain is healthy and functioning normally. But what if the feelings don't go away even though the tragic circumstances have passed or were a long time ago? It's possible that you're depressed.

Feeling depressed or sad can be a natural reaction to life's difficulties, losses, or damaged self-esteem. This is our brain "telling" us that something is wrong. However, if the brain "keeps telling" you that something is wrong when there isn't, it could be clinical depression. a medical condition that is both serious and treatable.

To summarize depression in a single sentence:

Extreme sadness, hopelessness, worthlessness, or helplessness that lasts for days, weeks, or even months

Every year, approximately 5 out of every 100 adults suffer from depression. Sometimes it only lasts a couple of weeks. However, one in every four women and one in every ten men will experience a depressive episode severe enough to necessitate treatment.

There are numerous factors that contribute to depression. A variety of physical conditions can increase your susceptibility to depression. Some people are genetically predisposed to pessimism and sadness. Depression can be caused by hormonal, neurological, or physical changes. Serious medical conditions such as chronic pain, heart disease, cancer, or HIV can also contribute to depression owing to the emotional stress they cause. In some cases, drugs used to treat medical conditions cause depression. Finally, depression can exacerbate health problems by weakening the immune system and making pain more difficult to bear.

Global changes are occurring at a faster rate than ever before in human history. The rate at which these changes are occurring is contributing to the largest increase in the number of people experiencing depression today. Many people are overwhelmed by the amount of pressure and anxiety they feel about the future. When your emotions are unable to keep up with everything, your emotional system becomes clogged and eventually signs off in resignation. When you give up on your creative life force, it quickly leads to depression and a slew of other problems.

Chronic depression causes biochemical and neurological imbalances that influence how you feel about yourself and how you think about things. A disease state keeps stress signals active between your heart and brain, altering the neurotransmitters and hormones released in your body and influencing your perceptions and moods. If those stress signals and neurochemical changes become constant, your brain believes this is your new normal state and resets to lock in the pattern. Then, no matter what you do, it's difficult to feel better. You can suffer in silence, seek comfort from friends, religion, or self-help methods, or try therapy or medication. Overwork or stimulants may be used to mask your distress. But the depression won't go away until you change your habits.

- Depression is a mental state in which a person feels completely empty, anxious, and lost. It is the lowest point on the emotional scale and is characterized by a wide range of negative emotions such as guilt, helplessness, anger, irritability, and so on.
- Depression is more than just a mood swing. It is a behavioral disorder that, like any other, requires treatment. Regardless of how happy a person is, depression must be treated.
- Depression is not the same as sadness. Sadness is a feeling. It is, without a doubt, painful and negative, but it is nowhere near as serious as depression.
- Depression can be caused by a number of factors. Some of the most common are traumatic childhood events, sexual abuse, family pressures, and so on. A loved one's death may also be a factor.
- Other reasons could include life-changing events such as childbirth, menopause, any medical diagnosis, and so on.
- The most common causes of depression in adolescents are societal rejection, bullying, peer pressure, and so on.

- Certain medications, such as Hepatitis C medication, sleep medication, high blood pressure medication, and so on, are also known to cause depression. Such instances are referred to as "medically induced depression."
- Substance abuse, such as with narcotics, is another major cause of depression.
- Dangerous behavior
- Suicidal thoughts, etc.
- Self-hatred or self-loathing
- Unexplained guilt and anger
- Crying for no apparent reason

Types of depression

There are two types of depression: **major** and **minor.**

1. **Major Depressive Disorder**

You will feel terrible or extremely sad for a few weeks, but this will pass. Major depression symptoms include loss of interest in life; feeling guilty for no apparent reason; suicidal thoughts; weight loss or gain; sleeping less or too much; being tired all the time; and difficulty concentrating. It is also associated with low self-esteem; people who have low self-esteem are more likely to suffer from major depression.

2. **Major Depressive Disorder (or dysthymia)**

It has the same symptoms as major depression, but the person suffers from it for at least two years.

This is a more severe form of major depression. It is extremely difficult for an individual to report this type of depression because the symptoms have become strong habits, and the individual believes "they have always been like this." Furthermore, it is more difficult for the individual's surroundings to recognize if the individual has this type of depression. The individual's surroundings will believe that this is the nature of his personality.

No matter how you look at it, if someone has negative thoughts or a negative mood for more than two weeks, you can almost certainly say that person is depressed.

Other Types Includes:

Dysthymia

Dysthymia is a type of depression that has mild symptoms overall, but these symptoms are chronic and can last for years. The following are the symptoms of this chronic state of mood:

You will be uninterested in daily activities, so you will be unmotivated to do anything.

Sadness Hopelessness

Insufficient energy

Being overly critical of oneself

Easily enraged. You might be easily irritated with friends and family.

Obsessing over your previous actions Sleeping difficulties

Being labeled as a pessimistic, gloomy person will be a frequent occurrence in your life.

These symptoms will stay with a person for years, but their intensity will fluctuate. As a result, you may have good and bad days. Though it is normal for bad days to last for months at a time with only a few good days in between.

Depressive Psychosis

This is a type of depression that is distinguished by a psychotic component. This means that, in addition to the classic depression symptoms, a person suffering from psychotic depression may hallucinate, such as hearing voices, or misinterpretations of reality, such as the belief that you are worthless or sinful.

Depression after childbirth

This is a type of depression experienced by mothers after giving birth. This mood shift can occur at any time during the first year after childbirth. It has been shown that approximately 10–15 percent of all new mothers will experience some form of postpartum depression, which can interfere with child rearing. These are the symptoms of this depressive disorder:

Appetite suppression

A feeling of resentment or hatred toward your child

The sexual drive has been lost.

A sense of inadequacy

A failure to connect with or bond with your child

Swings in mood: sleep deprivation

Leaving your husband, family, and friends Have you considered harming your child?

Seasonal Affective Disorder (SAD)

A person who feels blue during the long winter months may be suffering from SAD, or they may become depressed during the long, hot summer days.

The seasons have an impact on this type of depression. Seasonal affective disorder refers to any depressive mood that is triggered by the changing of the seasons. The specific symptoms you experience are determined by the season that's got you down.

Winter:

- A sense of heaviness Sleeping more frequently than usual
- Gaining weight and having cravings for fatty foods
- Irritability
- being unfriendly to people during the winter months. As a result, you may be irritable or snappy with family, friends, or even strangers.

Summer:

- Loss of weight
- Appetite loss

- Sleep deprivation
- Anxiety
- Sadness

Manic-depressive disorder or bipolar disorder

A person suffering from bipolar disorder may feel euphoric one moment and extremely depressed and unhappy the next. Bipolar disorder is distinguished by severe mood swings.

High mood symptoms include:

They will experience extreme happiness, even euphoria. You will feel fantastic about yourself.

Rapid-fire speech

Poor decision-making abilities quick to rage

Irritability

A rise in high-risk activity. This could include inappropriate sexual behavior, excessive drinking, or driving recklessly.

An increased interest in sex Motivation and ambition Spending with carelessness and not sleeping too much.

Mood symptoms include:

Unhappiness

A sense of foreboding about future appetite loss

The sexual drive has been lost.

Sleeping problems

Anxiety

There will be a lack of enjoyment in life.

Previously enjoyable hobbies will now be met with disinterest.

Irritability

Energy depletion

Depression in Childhood

It could be a normal emotion as your child grows. When your child is sad, it does not always imply that he or she is depressed. However, if your child is depressed on a daily basis, he or she may have a problem. Another sign is if the emotion interferes with his daily activities, such as schoolwork, family life, and hobbies.

Depression in Adolescents

When your teen is depressed for two weeks in a row, you should consult a doctor. They may be aloof when you speak to them, and they may not communicate well with their parents. They may also feel isolated and limit their contact with their friends. There are effective methods of treatment that are available to help you overcome depression. According to statistics, one out of every eight teenagers suffers from depression. This is a serious matter that must be dealt with properly.

Depression on two levels

This occurs when a person who is already suffering from chronic depression experiences trauma, which results in major depression.

Secondary Depressive Disorder

Depression caused by a known medical condition, such as Parkinson's disease, stroke, AIDS, or hypothyroidism It can also be caused by psychiatric disorders like panic disorder, bulimia, or schizophrenia.

Depression Refuses to Be Treated

This type of depression can be chronic or long-term.

This is a condition that does not respond well to antidepressant medications. Depending on the severity and nature of the condition, some suggest electroconvulsive therapy (ECT).

Depression with a Mask

This type of depression hides behind a person's physical complaints, and no cause can be identified.

Chapter 2
Symptoms of Depression

Several steps were taken to determine which symptoms should be included here. First, several psychiatric textbooks and monographs on depression were examined to determine which symptoms have been widely associated with depression. Second, I attempted to count which symptoms occurred significantly more frequently in the depressed group than in the non-depressed group in an intensive study of 50 depressed patients and 30 non-depressed patients in psychotherapy. Based on this tabulation, an inventory of depression-related items was created and pretested on approximately 100 patients. Finally, this questionnaire was revised and administered to 966 psychiatric patients.

One of the symptoms, irritability, was not significantly more common in depressed patients than in nondepressed patients. As a result, it has been removed from the list.

Some of the symptoms commonly associated with manic-depressive syndrome are not described in this chapter. For example, fear of death was not included because it was found to be no more common in depressed patients than in nondepressed patients in the preliminary clinical study. It was discovered that 42 percent of anxiety neurosis patients and only 35 percent of manic-depressive patients feared death. Similarly, 60 percent of manic-depressive patients and 54 percent of hysteria patients experienced constipation. As a result, this symptom does not appear to be unique to depression.

In our symptomatology analyses, we did not use conventional nosological categories. Rather than being classified based on their primary diagnoses, such as manic-depressive reactions, schizophrenia, anxiety reactions, and so on, the patients were classified based on the depth of depression they displayed, regardless of their primary diagnoses. This was due to two major factors. First, it was discovered in our own and previous studies that the degree of inter judge reliability in diagnoses made using standard nomenclature was relatively low. As a result, any findings based on diagnoses with such low reliability would be of questionable value. Inter psychiatrist ratings of depression depth, on the other hand, showed a relatively high correlation (.87). Second, we discovered that the cluster of symptoms commonly associated with the depressive syndrome occurs not only in disorders such as neurotic-depressive reaction and manic-depressive reaction but also in patients with anxiety reactions, schizophrenia, obsessional neurosis, and other conditions. In fact, we discovered that a patient with a primary diagnosis in one of the typical depressive categories may be less depressed than a patient with, say, schizophrenia or obsessional neurosis. As a result, the sample was divided into four groups based on the severity of the depression: none, mild, moderate, and severe.

I attempted to provide a guide for assessing the severity of the symptoms in addition to making the usual qualitative distinctions among them. The symptoms are discussed in terms of how they are likely to manifest themselves in the mild, moderate, and severe cases.

Depression level

Depression can be classified into mild, moderate, or severe states (or phases). This could help the clinician or researcher make a quantitative estimate of the severity of depression. The tables can be used to help with depression diagnosis because they show the relative frequency of symptoms in patients who were classified as nondepressed, mildly depressed, moderately depressed, or severely depressed.

Emotional Expressions

The term "emotional manifestations" refers to changes in the patient's feelings or overt behavior that are directly related to his or her emotional states. When assessing emotional manifestations, it is critical to consider the individual's premorbid mood and behavior, as well as what the examiner may consider the normal range for the patient's age, gender, and social group. A patient's occurrence of frequent crying spells who cried infrequently or never before becoming depressed may have a higher level of depression than a patient who cried infrequently, whether depressed or not.

Depressed Mood

Various clinically depressed patients describe the typical depression in mood in different ways. The examiner should investigate whatever term the patient uses to describe her or his subjective feelings. If the patient uses the word "depressed," for example, the examiner should not take it at face value but should try to figure out what it means for the patient. Individuals who are not clinically depressed may use this adjective to describe fleeting feelings of loneliness, boredom, or discouragement.

Sometimes the emotion is expressed primarily in somatic terms, such as "a lump in my throat," "an empty feeling in my stomach," or "a sad, heavy feeling in my chest." Further investigation reveals that these feelings are generally similar to those expressed by other patients in terms of adjectives such as sad, unhappy, lonely, or bored.

The examiner must assess the severity of the mood deviation. The relative degree or morbidity implied by the adjective chosen, the qualification by adverbs such as "slightly" or "very," and the degree of tolerance the patient expresses for the feeling (e.g., "I feel so miserable I can't stand it another minute") are some rough criteria for the degree of depression.

Among the adjectives used by depressed patients in response to the question "How do you feel?" are sad, lonely, unhappy, downhearted, humiliated, ashamed, worried, useless, and guilty. Eighty-eight percent of severely depressed patients reported sadness or unhappiness, compared to 23 percent of non-depressed patients.

Mild: The patient reports feeling down or sad. The unpleasant feeling fluctuates significantly throughout the day, and the patient may even feel cheerful at times. Outside stimuli, such as a compliment, a joke, or a favorable event, can also partially or completely alleviate the dysphoric feeling. The examiner can usually elicit a positive response with minimal effort or ingenuity. Patients at this level typically respond to jokes or humorous anecdotes with genuine amusement.

Moderate: The dysphoria is more pronounced and persistent. The patient's mood is less likely to be influenced by others' attempts to cheer him or her up, and any relief is only temporary. A diurnal variation is also frequently present: the dysphoria is usually worse in the morning and lessens as the day goes on.

Severe depression patients frequently express feelings of "hopelessness" or "miserability." Patients who are agitated frequently state that they are "worried." In our study, 70% of severely depressed patients stated that they were sad all the time and "couldn't snap out of that they were so sad that it was very painful, or that they couldn't stand it.

Negative Self-Evaluation

Patients who are depressed frequently express negative feelings about themselves. These feelings are similar to the general dysphoric feelings described above, but they are distinct in that they are directed specifically at the self. The patients appear to be able to distinguish between feelings of dislike for themselves and negative attitudes about themselves, such as "I am worthless." The frequency of self-dislike ranged from 37% in the nondepressed group to 86% in the severely depressed group.

Mild: Patients express dissatisfaction with themselves. This feeling is accompanied by thoughts such as "I've let everyone down.... I could have passed if I had tried harder."

Moderate: The feeling of self-dislike is more intense and may progress to disgust with oneself. This is usually accompanied by thoughts like "I'm a weakling. I don't do anything right. I'm no good."

Severe: Patients may come to despise themselves as a result of their feelings. "I'm a terrible person. I don't deserve to live." are examples of statements from this stage. "I'm despicable. I despise myself."

Reduced Gratification

Loss of gratification is so pervasive in depression that many patients regard it as the defining feature of their illness. In our study, 92 percent of severely depressed patients reported a loss of satisfaction. This was the most common symptom among all depressed people.

Loss of gratification appears to begin with a few activities and spread to almost everything the patient does as the depression progresses. Even activities associated with biological needs or drives, such as eating or sexual experiences, are not immune. Psychosocial experiences, such as achieving fame, receiving expressions of love or friendship, or even engaging in conversations, are similarly devoid of pleasurable properties.

Some patients' emphasis on their loss of satisfaction gives the impression that they are particularly oriented in their lives toward obtaining gratification. It is impossible to say whether or not this applies to the premorbid state, but it is true that the feverish pursuit of gratification is a key feature of their manic states.

The initial loss of satisfaction from activities involving responsibility or obligation, such as those associated with the roles of worker, stay-at-home spouse, or student, is frequently compensated for by increased satisfaction from recreational activities. This observation has led us to propose that, in depression, the "give-get" balance is disrupted: the patient, depleted psychologically over time by activities predominantly giving in nature, experiences an accentuation of passive needs, which are gratified by activities involving less of a sense of duty or responsibility (giving) and more of a tangible and easily gratifiable reward (reward) obtained fulfillment. However, in the later stages of the illness, even passive, regressive activities are ineffective.

Mild: The patient laments the loss of some of life's joy. He or she no longer derives pleasure or a "kick" from family, friends, or work. Activities involving responsibility, obligation, or effort become less satisfying over time. Patients frequently find more satisfaction in passive activities such as recreation, relaxation, or rest. They may seek out unusual activities in order to recapture some of their former thrills. One patient claimed that watching a performance of deviant sexual practices could always lift him out of a mild depression.

Moderate: Patients are frequently bored. They may try to engage in some of their previous favorite activities, but these now appear "flat." Business or professional activities that used to excite them no longer do. They may find temporary relief from a change, such as a vacation, but the boredom returns when normal activities are resumed.

Severe: They no longer enjoy previously pleasurable activities and may even develop an aversion to activities they once enjoyed. Popular acclaim or expressions of love or friendship no longer provide any level of fulfillment. Almost all of the patients complain that nothing gives them any satisfaction.

Loss of Emotional Attachment

Loss of emotional involvement in other people or activities is often associated with loss of satisfaction. This is manifested by a decrease in interest in specific activities as well as in affection for or concern for other people. Loss of affection for family members is frequently a source of concern for the patient, and it is occasionally a driving factor in seeking medical attention. Sixty-four percent of severely depressed patients reported a loss of feeling for or interest in other people, compared to only 16 percent of nondepressed patients.

Mild: In mild cases, there is a decrease in enthusiasm for or absorption in an activity. The patient may report that they no longer feel the same intensity of love or affection for their spouse, children, or friends, but they may also feel more dependent on them.

Moderate: Loss of interest or positive feelings can lead to indifference. A number of patients described it as a "wall" between them and others. A husband may complain that he no longer loves his wife, or a mother may be concerned that she appears to care little about her children or what happens to them. A previously devoted employee may report that he or she is no longer concerned about his or her job. Both men and women may have lost interest in their physical appearance.

Severe: Apathy may develop as a result of the loss of attachment to external objects. The patient may not only lose any positive feelings for family members but he or she may be surprised to discover that their only reaction is negative. In some cases, the patient only feels cold hatred, which may be masked by dependency. "I've been told I have love and can give love," says a typical patient. But now I have no feelings for my family. I couldn't care less about them. "I know it's terrible, but I sometimes despise them."

Crying Fits

Depressed patients frequently cry for extended periods of time. This is especially true for the women in our series who are depressed. Eighty-three percent of severely depressed patients reported crying more frequently than they did before becoming depressed or feeling like crying even if the tears did not come.

Some patients who cried infrequently when they were not depressed were able to detect the onset of depression by observing a strong desire to cry. "I don't know whether I'm sad or not, but I feel like crying, so I guess I'm depressed," one woman said. Further probing revealed the remaining cardinal symptoms of depression.

Mild: There is an increased proclivity to cry or weep. Stimuli or situations that would not normally affect the patient may now cause tears. A mother, for example, may cry during an argument with her children or if she believes her husband is not paying attention. Although mildly depressed women frequently cry, it is unusual for a mildly depressed man to do so.

Moderate: During the psychiatric interview, the patient may cry, and references to his or her problems may cause tears. Men who haven't cried since childhood may cry as they talk about their problems. "It just comes over me like a wave, and I can't stop crying," say some women. Patients may feel relieved after crying, but they are more likely to feel depressed.

Severe: Patients who were easily moved to tears in the earlier stages may find that they can no longer cry even when they want to by the time they reach the severe stage. They may cry but do not shed tears ("dry depression"); Although they had previously been capable of crying, 29 percent reported that they couldn't cry when they were sad, even though they wanted to.

Response to loss of laughter

Depressed patients frequently reveal that they have lost their sense of humor. The issue does not appear to be a loss of ability to perceive the point of the joke or even to construct a joke when instructed. The problem appears to be that patients do not respond to humor in a typical way. They are not amused, do not want to laugh, and receive no satisfaction from a sarcastic remark, joke, or cartoon.

In our study, 52 percent of severely depressed patients said they had lost their sense of humor, compared to 8 percent of nondepressed patients.

Mild: Patients who frequently enjoy listening to and telling jokes discover that this is no longer such an easy source of pleasure. They express their dissatisfaction with jokes.

Furthermore, they do not tolerate teasing or joking from their friends as well as they did previously.

Moderate: Patients may understand the gist of a joke and even try to smile, but they are rarely amused. They are unable to see the humor in events and tend to take everything seriously.

Severe: Patients do not respond to other people's amusing remarks. Whereas others may laugh at the humorous element of a joke, they are more likely to be hurt or disgusted by the aggressive or hostile content.

Cognitive Significance

Depression's cognitive manifestations include a wide range of symptoms. The patient's distorted attitudes toward self, personal experience, and the future comprise one group. This category includes low self-esteem, body image distortions, and negative expectations. Another symptom, self-blame, expresses patients' understanding of causality: they are inclined to blame themselves for any difficulties or problems they encounter. The third type of symptom concerns decision-making. Typically, the patient vacillates and is indecisive.

Low Self-Evaluation

Depression is characterized by low self-esteem. Self-devaluation appears to be part of the pattern of depressed patients viewing themselves as lacking in specific attributes that are important to them: ability, performance, intelligence, health, strength, personal attractiveness, popularity, or financial resources. "I am inferior" or "I am inadequate" are common expressions of a sense of deficiency. This symptom was reported by 81% of severely depressed patients and 38% of those who were not depressed.

Complaints of a lack of love or material possessions may also reflect a sense of deficiency. This reaction is most noticeable in patients who have recently experienced an unhappy love affair or a financial setback.

Mild: Patients have an exaggerated reaction to their mistakes or difficulties and are prone to viewing them as a reflection of inadequacy or a flaw. They compare themselves to others and, more often than not, conclude that they are inferior. However, these inaccurate self-evaluations can be corrected, at least temporarily, by confronting patients with appropriate evidence or reasoning with them.

Moderate: The majority of patients' thought content revolves around a sense of deficiency, and they are prone to misinterpreting neutral situations as evidence of this deficiency. They exaggerate the magnitude and significance of any mistakes. When they reflect on their current and past lives, their failures stand out and their successes pale in comparison. They complain that they have lost confidence in themselves, and their sense of inadequacy is such that when confronted with tasks that they have easily handled in the past, their first thought is, "I can't do it."

Patients who are religious or moralistic tend to dwell on their sins or moral failings. Patients who place a high value on personal attractiveness, intelligence, or business success believe they have deteriorated in these areas. Attempts to change patients' distorted self-evaluations by reassuring them or presenting contradictory evidence are generally met with considerable resistance; any increase in realistic thinking about themselves is transient.

Severe: Patients' self-evaluations are at an all-time low. They drastically reduce their personal attributes as well as their roles as parent, spouse, employer, and so on. They see themselves as worthless, inept, and total failures. They claim they are a burden to their family members and would do better without them. The severely depressed patient may be obsessed with being the world's worst sinner, completely impoverished, or completely inadequate. Attempts to correct incorrect ideas are usually futile.

Expectations that are negative

A bleak outlook and pessimism are closely related to the previously mentioned feelings of hopelessness. More than 78 percent of depressed patients had a negative outlook, compared to 22 percent of nondepressed patients. This symptom had the strongest relationship with the clinical rating of depression.

The pattern of depressed patients expecting the worst and rejecting the possibility of any improvement creates formidable barriers to engaging them in a therapeutic program. When friends, family, and physicians try to assist them, their negative outlook is often a source of frustration. Patients may, for example, throw away their antidepressant pills because they believe they "cannot do any good."

Unlike anxious patients, who temper negative expectations with the realization that the unpleasant events can be avoided or will pass in time, depressed patients envision a future in which the current deficient condition (financial, social, or physical) will persist or worsen. This sense of the permanency and irreversibility of one's situation or problems appears to be the foundation for contemplating suicide as a logical course of action. The finding that, of all the symptoms correlated with suicide, hopelessness had the highest correlation coefficient with suicide indicates the relationship between hopelessness and suicide.

In ambiguous or equivocal situations, patients tend to expect a negative outcome. When associates and friends feel justified in expecting positive outcomes, their expectations tend to be negative or pessimistic. Whether the issue is health, personal problems, or economic problems, they are skeptical that anything will change.

Moderate: They see the future as unpromising and claim to have nothing to look forward to. It is difficult to persuade them to do anything because their initial reaction is "I won't like it" or "it won't help."

They see the future as bleak and hopeless. They claim that they will never be able to overcome their difficulties and that things will never get better. They believe that none of their problems are solvable. They say things like, "This is the end of the road." "From now on, I will appear older and there's nothing here for me anymore. I have nowhere to go. "There is no future"; "I know I can't improve... it's all over for me."

Self-criticism and self-blame

The persistence of depressives' self-blame and self-criticism appears to be related to their egocentric notions of causality and proclivity for criticizing themselves for alleged deficiencies. They are especially prone to attribute negative events to some flaw in themselves and then chastise themselves for this alleged flaw. In more severe cases, patients may blame themselves for events that have nothing to do with them and abuse themselves brutally. This symptom was reported by 80% of severely depressed patients.

Mild: When patients fall short of their rigid, perfectionist standards, they are prone to blaming and criticizing themselves. People are more likely to berate themselves for being dull or stupid if they appear less responsive to them or take longer to solve a problem. They appear to be intolerant of any flaws in themselves and refuse to accept the notion that it is human to make mistakes. Moderate: Patients are likely to harshly criticize themselves for any aspects of their personality or behavior that they judge to be subpar. They are prone to blaming themselves for mistakes that are clearly not their fault. Their self-criticism becomes harsher.

Severe: Patients in the severe state are more extreme in their self-blame or self-criticism. They make statements like, "I am responsible for the world's violence and suffering." There is no way I can be punished sufficiently for my sins. "I wish you'd drag me out and hang me." They see themselves as social outcasts or criminals and interpret various external stimuli as indications of public disapproval.

Indecisiveness

Difficulty making decisions, vacillating between alternatives, and changing decisions are all depressive symptoms that can be frustrating for both the patient's family and friends. Indecisiveness was reported by 48 percent of mildly depressed patients and 76 percent of severely depressed patients.

This indecision appears to have at least two components. The first is primarily cognitive in nature. Depressed patients anticipate making the wrong choice: whenever they consider one of several options, they tend to regard it as incorrect and believe they will regret making that choice. The second facet is primarily motivational and is associated with "will paralysis," avoidance tendencies, and increased dependency. Patients are unmotivated to go through the mental operations required to reach a conclusion. Also, deciding represents a burden; they want to avoid or, at the very least, get help with any situation they perceive will be burdensome. Furthermore, they recognize that deciding frequently commits them to a course of action, and because they want to avoid action, they procrastinate.

Routine decisions that must be made in order to carry out their occupational or household responsibilities become major issues for depressed patients. A professor cannot decide what material to include in a lecture; a housewife cannot decide what to cook for dinner; a student cannot decide whether to spend the spring break studying at college or at home, and an executive cannot decide whether to hire a new assistant.

Mild: Patients who can normally make quick decisions find that solutions do not come as easily. Whereas in their normal state they plan "without even thinking about it," they now feel compelled to ponder the issue, consider the potential consequences of the decision, and consider a variety of often irrelevant alternatives. A general sense of uncertainty reflects the fear of making the wrong decision. They frequently seek confirmation from another person.

Moderate: Decision-making difficulty extends to almost every activity and includes minor issues such as what clothes to wear, which route to take to work, and whether to get a haircut. It is often immaterial which alternative is chosen, but hesitating and failing to make a decision can have negative consequences. A woman, for example, spent several weeks deciding between two paint colors for her home. The two shades under consideration were barely distinguishable, but her inability to decide caused a commotion in the house, with the painter abandoning his buckets of paint and scaffolding until a decision could be made.

Severe: Depressed patients generally believe they are incapable of making decisions and, as a result, do not even attempt to do so. When asked to make a shopping list or a list of clothes for her children to bring to camp, a woman insisted she couldn't decide what to write down. Patients frequently question everything they do and say. One woman was skeptical that she had given the psychiatrist her correct name and pronounced it correctly.

Body image distortion

In depression, patients' distorted perceptions of their physical appearance are frequently quite noticeable. This occurs slightly more frequently in women than in men. In our study, 66 percent of severely depressed patients believed they had lost their attractiveness, compared to 12 percent of nondepressed patients.

Mild: Patients become overly concerned with their physical appearance. Every time she passes a mirror, a woman frowns at her reflection. She scrutinizes her face for blemishes and becomes preoccupied with the notion that she looks plain or is gaining weight. A man is constantly concerned about the onset of hair loss, convinced that women find him unattractive.

Moderate: Concerns about physical appearance are more prevalent. A man believes that his appearance has changed since the onset of his depression, despite the fact that there is no objective evidence to support this belief. When he sees someone who is ugly, he thinks to himself, "I look like that." His brow furrows as he becomes concerned about his appearance. When he looks in the mirror at his furrowed brow, he thinks, "My whole face is wrinkled, and the wrinkles will never go away." Some patients seek plastic surgery to correct distorted or exaggerated facial features.

Even if there is no objective evidence, a woman may believe she has gained weight. In fact, some patients believe this even when they are losing weight.

Severe: The concept of personal unattractiveness becomes more firmly established. Patients believe they are repulsive and ugly. They anticipate that others will turn away in disgust; one woman wore a veil, and another turned her head whenever anyone approached her.

Chapter 3
Manifestations of Motivation

In depression, motivational manifestations include consciously experienced strivings, desires, and impulses. These motivational patterns are frequently inferred from observing the patient's behavior; however, direct questioning usually elicits a fairly precise and comprehensive description of motivation.

The regressive nature of the depressed patient's characteristic motivations is a striking feature. The term "regressive" refers to the patient's tendency to gravitate toward activities that require the least amount of responsibility, initiative, or energy. They avoid activities that are specifically associated with the adult role in favor of activities that are more typical of the child's role. When given a choice, they prefer passivity to activity and dependence to independence (autonomy); they avoid responsibility and seek to avoid rather than solve their problems; they seek immediate but fleeting gratifications rather than delayed but prolonged satisfactions. The ultimate manifestation of the escapist trend is the desire to commit suicide in order to escape life.

One crucial aspect of these motivations is that their fulfillment is typically incompatible with the individual's major premorbid goals and values. In essence, giving in to passive impulses and desires to withdraw or commit suicide results in the abandonment of family, friends, and vocation. Similarly, the patient passes up the opportunity to gain personal fulfillment through accomplishment.

or interpersonal interactions Furthermore, by avoiding even the simplest problems, the patient discovers that they accumulate until they appear overwhelming.

The specific motivational patterns to be described are presented as separate phenomena, despite the fact that they are obviously interconnected and may represent different facets of the same fundamental pattern. It is possible that some phenomena are primary while others are secondary or tertiary; for example, it is possible that paralysis of the will is caused by escapist or passive desires, a sense of futility, a loss of external investments, or a sense of fatigue. Because these suggestions are purely speculative, it appears preferable to treat these phenomena separately for the time being rather than prematurely assigning primacy to certain patterns.

Willpower paralysis

The loss of positive motivation is a common symptom of depression. Patients may struggle to mobilize themselves to perform even the most basic and essential tasks, such as eating, eliminating waste, or taking medication to relieve their distress. The essence of the problem appears to be that, while they can define what they should do for themselves, they do not experience any internal stimulus to do it. Even when pressed, cajoled, or threatened, they do not appear to be motivated to do these things. Positive motivation was lost in 65 percent of mild cases and 86 percent of severe cases.

An actual or impending change in a patient's life situation may occasionally serve to mobilize constructive motivations. One particularly retarded and apathetic patient was aroused when her husband became ill, and she felt compelled to assist him. Another patient experienced a resurgence of positive motivation after learning she would be hospitalized, a prospect she despised.

Mild: Patients notice that they no longer have a spontaneous desire to do certain things, particularly those that do not provide immediate gratification. An advertising executive notices a loss of drive and initiative in planning a special sales promotion; a college professor loses interest in preparing his lectures, and a medical student loses interest in studying. A retiree who used to be motivated to participate in a variety of domestic and community projects described her lack of motivation as follows: "I have no desire to do anything." I just go through the motions with no regard for what I'm doing. "I just go through the motions like a robot, and when I run out of energy, I simply stop."

Moderate: In moderate cases, the loss of spontaneous desire spreads to almost all of the patient's usual activities. "There are certain things I know I have to do, like eat, brush my teeth, and go to the bathroom, but I have no desire to do them," said one woman. In contrast to the severely depressed patients, particularly moderately depressed patients, discover that they can "force" themselves to do things. They are also sensitive to peer pressure and potentially embarrassing situations. A woman, for example, stood in front of an elevator for about 15 minutes because she couldn't bring herself to press the button. When others approached the elevator, she quickly pressed the button so they wouldn't think she was strange.

Severe: In severe cases, the will is frequently paralyzed. Patients have no desire to do anything, even things that are necessary for survival. As a result, unless prodded or pushed into activity by others, they may be relatively immobile. Patients must sometimes be dragged out of bed, washed, dressed, and fed. In extreme cases, the patient's inertia may prevent communication. One woman, who was unable to respond to questions during the worst of her depression, later stated that even though she "wanted" to, she couldn't muster the "willpower" to do so.

Wishes for Avoidance, Escapism, and Withdrawal

The desire to break free from one's usual pattern or routine is a common symptom of depression. The office assistant wishes to be free of paperwork, the student fantasizes about faraway places, and the stay-at-home spouse wishes to be free of domestic duties. Depressed people see their responsibilities as dull, meaningless, or burdensome, and they want to escape to an activity that provides relaxation or refuge.

These escapist desires are similar to the attitudes described as having paralysis. Escapist wishes are experienced as definite motivations with specific goals, whereas "paralysis of the will" refers to a loss or absence of motivation.

Mild: mildly depressed patients have a strong desire to avoid or postpone doing things they find uninteresting or taxing. They tend to avoid attending to details that they consider unimportant. They are more likely to put off or avoid an activity that does not provide immediate gratification or requires effort. They are repelled by activities that require effort or responsibility, but they are drawn to more passive and simple activities.

"It's much easier to daydream in lectures than pay attention," said a depressed student. It's more convenient to stay at home and drink than to call a girl for a date. It's easier to mumble and go unnoticed than it is to speak clearly and distinctly. It's much easier to write sloppily than it is to write legibly. "It's much easier to live a self-centered, passive life than it is to try to change it."

Moderate: In moderate cases, avoidance desires are stronger and extend to a broader range of everyday activities. "Escape seems to be my strongest desire," said a depressed college professor. I have the impression that despite the fact that I would be happier in almost any other occupation or profession, "I wish I was a bus driver instead of a teacher as I ride the bus to university." Patients are constantly thinking of ways to distract themselves or escape. They prefer passive recreation such as going to the movies, watching television, or getting drunk. They may fantasize about visiting a desert island or becoming nomads. They may withdraw from most social contacts at this point because interpersonal relationships appear to be too demanding. At the same time, because of their loneliness and increased reliance, they may desire to interact with others.

Severe: In severe cases, the desire to avoid or escape manifests itself in extreme secrecy. The patient frequently remains in bed and, when approached, may hide under the covers. "I just feel like getting away from everybody and everything," said one patient. I'm not interested in seeing anyone or doing anything. "I just want to sleep." Suicide is a common form of escape for severely depressed patients.

They have a strong desire to end their lives in order to escape an unbearable situation.

Suicidal Thoughts

Suicidal thoughts have historically been associated with depression. Suicidal thoughts can occur in nondepressed people, but they are significantly more common in depressed patients. This was the symptom reported least frequently (12%) by non-depressed patients in our study, but it was reported frequently (74%) by severely depressed patients. This distinction highlights the diagnostic utility of this specific symptom in the detection of severe depression. The severity of this symptom was also found to have one of the strongest correlations with the severity of depression.

Suicidal ideation in a patient can manifest itself in a variety of ways. It can manifest as a passive wish ("I wish I were dead"), an activity wish ("I want to kill myself"), a repetitive, obsessive thought with no volitional quality, a daydream, or a meticulously conceived plan. Suicidal thoughts may occur in some patients throughout the illness, and the patient may have to fight them off constantly. In other cases, the wish is sporadic and characterized by a gradual build-up followed by a slackening of intensity until it temporarily disappears. Patients frequently express regret that they did not grant the wish after it had passed. It should be noted that an impulsive suicide attempt can be just as dangerous as a planned suicide attempt.

Suicidal symptoms are obviously important because they are currently the only feature of depression that has a reasonably high risk of fatal consequences. Suicide attempts among manic-depressives 2.8 percent in one study with a 10-year follow-up and 12 to 5% over a 25-year period of observation.

Mild: Around 31% of mildly depressed patients expressed a desire to die. These are frequently expressed in the passive form, such as "I'd be better off dead." Patients may claim that they would not do anything to hasten death, but they find the prospect of dying appealing. Because of the possibility of a plane crash, one patient looked forward to an airplane trip.

Sometimes the patient expresses apathy toward life ("I don't care if I live or die"). Other patients may exhibit ambivalence ("I want to die, but I'm afraid of dying").

Suicidal thoughts are more direct, frequent, and compelling in these cases, and there is a clear risk of either impulsive or premeditated suicidal attempts. This desire can be expressed passively: "I hope I don't wake up in the morning" or "If I died, my family would be better off." The active expression of the wish can range from the ambiguous, "I'd like to kill myself but I don't have the guts," to the blatant, "If I could do it and not mess it up, I would go ahead and kill myself." Suicidal thoughts can manifest themselves as the patient taking unnecessary risks. A number of patients drove at excessive speeds in the hope that something would happen.

Severe: In severe cases, suicidal thoughts are often intense, but the patient may be too retarded to complete a suicide attempt. Typical statements include the following: "I'm so hopeless," she says, "why don't you let me die? "Everything has been lost. "There is only one way out—I must commit suicide"; "I must weep myself to death." "I can't live, and you won't let me die"; "I can't bear another day." "Please put an end to my misery."

Chapter 4
Causes of Depression

A variety of factors can contribute to the development of depression. It is usually the result of several events, personal factors, and other long-term factors, rather than a single event.

According to studies, ongoing difficulties, such as being in an abusive relationship, long-term unemployment, prolonged exposure to work-related stress, or long-term loneliness, are more likely to cause depression than recent life events. Recent negative events, or a combination of these events and other factors, can, however, trigger depression in people who are already on edge due to personal factors or bad experiences.

The following are some of the factors that may contribute to depression:

Personality

Some people are more likely to suffer from depression because they are perfectionists, worry excessively, lack self-esteem, are pessimists, or are sensitive to criticism.

Ancestral history

People who have a family history of depression are more likely to suffer from it. However, having a depressed parent or close relative does not automatically make you depressed. Other personal factors and circumstances will likely determine whether or not you will experience depression.

Abuse of drugs and alcohol

This can contribute to or cause depression. Many people who are depressed also have drug and/or alcohol problems.

Serious Medical Conditions

Medical illnesses can either directly cause depression or trigger it through stress and worry, particularly if the condition involves chronic pain or long-term management.

Conflict

Personal conflicts or fights with family members or friends are frequently the cause of conflict depression in biologically vulnerable people.

Certain medications

Corticosteroids, the antiviral drug interferon-alpha, and Accutane are examples of medications that may increase a person's risk of depression.

Death or loss

Overwhelming grief or sadness caused by the death of a loved one may increase a person's risk of depression.

Significant occurrences

Graduation, a new job, or even marriage can all lead to depression, as can job loss, relocation, retirement, or divorce. These are events that some people may find difficult to deal with, especially because they bring about major changes.

Other personal issues

Depression can be triggered by mental illnesses, social isolation, or being an outcast.

Despite the fact that depression is very common, it is frequently misdiagnosed or ignored. However, ignoring it can lead to life-threatening situations, especially since severe depression is linked to a high suicide rate. Early detection and awareness can help you find qualified help. If you or a loved one begins to exhibit symptoms of depression, seek help immediately.

Chapter 5
Treatment for Depression

After you've admitted that you have depression, the next step is to figure out how to get rid of it. There are three approaches to treating depression that you can take: medication, therapy, and lifestyle changes.

Medication

If you decide to seek help from a medical professional for your depression, they may advise you to take antidepressants. Antidepressants can be used to treat clinical depression, seasonal affective disorder (SAD), and dysthymia. There are several types of antidepressants that can help alleviate the symptoms of depression. Selective serotonin reuptake inhibitors, or SSRIs, are the most commonly prescribed class of medication.

These work by increasing the levels of serotonin and noradrenaline in the brain, which are two chemicals that influence mood. Citalopram, Paroxetine, Zoloft, Lexapro, Prozac, Cymbalta, Venlafaxine, and Luvox are examples of commonly prescribed antidepressants.

However, it is important to remember that there are a few negative side effects that can occur while taking antidepressants. They are as follows:

Nausea Fatigue

Loss of sexual interest

Anxiety levels have risen.

Restlessness

Dizziness

Gained weight

Dry mouth

Changes in bowel habits

Headaches

Sweating excessively

Suicidal ideation has increased.

The majority of these side effects should subside within three weeks of starting antidepressants.

Antidepressants are not addictive, but they can cause problems if you suddenly stop taking them. To stop taking this type of medication, you must first consult with a medical professional. He or she will devise a safe plan to gradually wean you off of them with minimal side effects.

The effects felt if you stop taking antidepressants abruptly, you may experience a slew of unpleasant side effects. These are:

Nausea, headaches, anxiety, and vomiting

Mood swings that are extreme Insomnia

Dizziness when easily enraged

Coordination problems

shocks to the brain. a strange sensation that feels like your brain is being shocked. These shocks can sometimes be felt in other parts of the body.

The tremors

A different treatment method, hospitalization, will be required for psychosis-related depression. While in the hospital, the patient will receive proper care and support, as well as medication in the form of antidepressants and antipsychotic medications, which will aid in the cessation of hallucinations.

Natural vs. Pharmaceutical Treatment

Depression, like any other disease of the mind and psyche, is easily treatable in a variety of ways.

Ideas on how to combat depression took center stage in the nineteenth century, coinciding with the medical breakthroughs and economic advancements of the time.

Many blamed the Industrial Revolution, with its factories and workshops, for creating an environment in which people felt alienated and insignificant. Nonetheless, scientists have reason to believe that certain biological processes and physical world factors influence the onset of depression.

Today, however, experts are using both natural and synthetic methods to treat depression. However, there appears to be a conflict between the two, a conflict that should determine which method to use.

We're trying to weigh our options here.

Depression vs. drugs

Your local pharmacy may stock a wide range of medications designed specifically for the treatment of depression. Indeed, modern innovations have contributed to the development of medications that aid in the treatment of such psychological disorders.

Antidepressants are widely available in pharmacies. Specific types of these drugs, however, are heavily regulated due to the significant psycho-physical changes they cause.

Often, tricyclic antidepressants are the most effective. These medications work by influencing two chemical messengers that influence depression, namely serotonin and norepinephrine.

Doctors, on the other hand, frequently prescribe selective serotonin reuptake inhibitors. These antidepressants are known to be safe and well tolerated by the majority of people.

Reversible inhibitors of monoamine oxidase are commonly used as substitutes for other types of antidepressants for people who have difficulty sleeping because they have fewer side effects. However, these are thought to be far less effective in terms of influencing the amount of neurotransmitters that cause depression.

Most pharmacies now stock newer antidepressant medications. Noradrenaline-Serotonin-Specific Antidepressants are widely available. The promise of minimal side effects is no reason to rely solely on these drugs. Weight gain and changes in sexual appetite can be harmful.

These medications have been shown to be effective in treating depression. However, you will still need to seek medical advice before proceeding with the use of these drugs, which we can all assume are not cheap.

Natural Method

With consistent medication, you may as well take the natural route to depression treatment. Keep in mind that, while drugs are known to be effective, they can also irritate certain aspects of your lifestyle. and reliance may be the least of your concerns.

As a result, your best bet is to base your treatment on emotions; anything that can bring you comfort.

Natural alternatives include activities like learning a new hobby or talking with someone close to you.

People have different ways of dealing with sadness, and it all depends on whether you want to be saved from this melancholy pit or not.

However, not everyone can say that dealing with depression is easy.

Chapter 6
Reasons for being SAD

Many patients suffering from depression are unsure how they became depressed. Others would deny the source or causes of their sadness until they were able to tolerate their depression.

We have learned that the factors that cause depression can be both physical and emotional. To take a materialist approach, it is possible that chemical interactions within your body influence moods and thought processes, but this has yet to be proven in medical and academic circles.

With that in mind, there is only one source of clarity: the individual.

What's the matter with you?

Patients frequently report being confronted by negative thoughts or memories that remind them of traumatic experiences or merely significant life events.

According to studies, nearly all people suffering from depression have no idea why they are suffering in the first place, adding to the human mind's enigma.

But if we could tap into certain aspects of a patient's thoughts, his whims and desires, and his musings, we might be able to get close to the root of the depression and find the best treatment for it.

Conversation as a Treatment

The procedure is straightforward. When you are depressed, you are usually interrogated by a clinical psychiatry expert. Most patients, however, prefer not to give honest opinions about themselves, instead trying to mislead their interviewers with hazy answers and exaggerated anecdotes.

Most patients would prefer not to express themselves. It is more likely that they believe their depression will be incurable for an indefinite period of time or that they are so depressed that any attempt at social interaction is considered taboo.

Yes, it can be a difficult task at times, but this method allows you to clear your mind of anything that may be contributing to your depressed feelings of worthlessness and distrust. Your therapist is here to help you.

This is a process that you must trust, and you can only hope that by sharing your true feelings and resisting the urge to suppress them, you will gradually relieve yourself of the burden of sadness.

The importance of expression

Being depressed is not an excuse to isolate yourself. On the bright side, you can take advantage of your solitude. It allows you to evaluate certain aspects of your life and determine which of them bother you the most. Is it possible that people have become too superficial for you? Were there events in your past that contributed to your current situation?

Try to be truthful to yourself. Your depression did not appear out of nowhere, and we cannot simply assume that it was caused by the actions of certain hormones in your body. Perhaps there are aspects of your life that require careful reflection, which can only be accomplished when you choose to stop crying and confront the realms of your life.

Counseling or therapy

This type of treatment, which can be done alongside or instead of medication, entails discussing issues or concerns that make you unhappy. The most important decision you will need to make regarding this type of treatment is who you will be speaking with. To begin, ask your doctor for a list of recommended therapists or counselors. Next, schedule appointments with several of the names on the list. Meet with them to discuss your feelings about them. Do they make you feel at ease? Or, conversely, do they make you feel awkward and uncomfortable? In addition, consider the location of the therapy. Is it warm and inviting, or sterile and icy? Find a location and a person who will provide the most supportive environment. If this means meeting with a variety of people until you find the right one, so be it. This is about you and your attempt to free yourself from the deliberate sadness you've become trapped within.

Therapy can help alleviate depression for a variety of reasons. It can be extremely therapeutic to talk about issues in your life that have caused you grief or stress, such as a divorce or a family death. Therapy can also provide coping strategies for depression and attempt to change certain thought patterns or behaviors, such as learning not to be so harsh on yourself.

Seek assistance or speak with someone.

As previously stated, seeking help from friends and loved ones can assist you in overcoming depression.

Social relations serve purposes other than utility. We can certainly rely on our parents or friends for certain things, such as money or favors. However, the emotional attachment to these relationships is what defines the human experience.

And, having known you for a long time, your friends and family can certainly serve as emotional walls for you to lean on when sadness overwhelms you. To do so, you must first recognize the need to overcome social anxiety. Communication is essential and a genuine human need, and you will undoubtedly need to practice it in order to confront the sadness.

Friendly Suggestions

Your friends can very well serve as your trusted confidants.

You and I have been friends for a long time. You've been to hell and back, forming a kind of brotherly or sisterly bond. And you'd gladly give each other advice on just about anything.

If the going gets tough as your depression worsens, the best thing you can do is ask your friends for help. They've known you for a long time, and seeing you depressed would be unusual for them, given that they've never seen you feel this way before.

Share your feelings with your friends. It's possible that your depression was brought on by a sense of alienation or simply the feeling that you're always left out.

Because they are familiar with your point of view, your friends may be able to offer you useful advice.

Family Counseling

In addition to friends, your family may have suggestions for how to alleviate your loneliness. Your parents, having seen how you have grown over time, would use their wisdom to solve your problems, whatever form they take.

Your parents, in their protective role, would feel empathy for you. You may have had a difficult time at school or at work. A recent divorce or break-up may have left you devastated. In such cases, you require some sort of clarity, something that can shed a rational light on your situation. Your parents can also teach you how to deal with emotional blocks by bringing their own experiences into the conversation.

Try to be open with your siblings as well. They might as well be concerned about what their sibling is going through.

Expert Opinion

You can, however, always seek the advice of experts in the study of human emotions and the psychological and biological forces at work.

Consult with a local psychiatrist. It may cost a lot of money to pay for the sessions and medication, but it can help in the long run, especially if the depression is deeply rooted in the psyche.

Chapter 7
Effects of Depression

Depression has an impact on one's physical well-being. Here are some of the physical consequences of depression:

1. Two out of every three people suffer from aches and pains.
2. Day-to-day exhaustion
3. Reduced libido
4. Periodic sleep deprivation, insomnia, or oversleeping When the brain wires incorrectly, serotonin deficiency occurs. Chronically depressed people are more sensitive to pain. Back pain is a common complaint among them. Depressed people's sexual lives are also influenced by serotonin. Relationships can suffer as a result of depression.

Unfortunately, many people suffering from depression, as well as their families and doctors, fail to recognize the warning signs. In one case, people who were found fatigued and suffering from insomnia were dismissed as simply aging when, in fact, they were depressed.

Depression and physical illness

Cortisol levels rise when you are stressed, increasing your risk of several diseases. It can harm your body by attacking your immune system. If this happens, you will be unable to fight infection. Even if you have been vaccinated, the effect is no longer as strong. There is also evidence that depression leads to drug abuse.

Depression and Medical Conditions

Physical challenges imposed on a person suffering from depression are said to weaken their immune system. As a result, pre-existing illnesses may worsen. Physical changes caused by depression or illness may precipitate or worsen depression.

The following serious illnesses are linked to depression:
Stroke

The heart attack

Coronary Artery Disease (CAD) Lupus Parkinson's disease (PD) or Multiple Sclerosis (MS)Cancer

HIV/AIDS

Diabetes

Kidney disease.

Arthritis

Depression may increase the risk of these diseases, but there is no direct link.

Chapter 8
Stress-Relieving Foods

You can try eating nutrient-rich foods to alleviate depression. However, there is no real link between what types of food help people who are depressed. Still, there is reason to believe that a well-balanced diet will meet the needs of people suffering from depression.

A healthy diet and good nutrition are essential in our daily lives. Omega-3, vitamin D, magnesium, vitamin B complex, folate, amino acids, iron, zinc, iodine, and selenium deficiencies are strongly linked to depression. However, a high intake of processed sugar, saturated fat, and trans fats is thought to contribute to depression. When you eat a lot of these foods, you are not providing your body and brain with the nutrition they require to function properly. To maximize your mood every day, eat balanced and healthy meals and avoid all processed sugars, saturated fats, and trans fats.

Consume nutrient-rich foods.

Nutrient-dense foods promote body growth, repair, and wellness. Everyone requires vitamins, carbohydrates, protein, and minerals. A little fat in one's diet wouldn't hurt. If you do not consume enough nutrients, your body will not function properly and may even become ill.

Your plate should contain antioxidants.

Normal body functions generate free radicals, which contribute to dysfunction and aging. Free radicals are combated by antioxidants. Consume foods that are high in vitamin C, beta-carotene, and vitamin E. According to research, free radicals endanger the brain. These foods can help you avoid free radicals:

Broccoli, apricots, carrots, cantaloupe, peaches, collards, spinach, sweet potatoes, and pumpkin are all high in beta-carotene.

Vitamin C-rich foods include broccoli, grapefruit, blueberries, oranges, peppers, and kiwis. Potatoes, tomatoes, and strawberries

Vitamin E-rich foods include seeds and nuts, vegetable oils, wheat germ, and margarine.

Eat the "right carbs" to reduce stress.

Serotonin, the "feel-good hormone," is linked to carbohydrates. According to one study, craving carbohydrates lowers serotonin levels. With this information, making smart carbohydrate choices, such as avoiding sugary foods, cookies, and cakes, may be the best option.

Consume protein to boost alertness.

Tyrosine is found in proteins such as chicken, tuna, and turkey. This amino acid increases the levels of dopamine and neopinephrine in your brain. It makes you feel alive and provides you with enough energy to stay alert and focused. Protein should be included in your diet on a daily basis.

Lean beef, peas and beans, low-fat cheese, milk, fish, yogurt, soy products, and poultry are all high in protein.

Yes, eat and drink liberally!

Following our discussion of foods that can depress your mood, here is a list of foods that can improve it. You should definitely try the following foods:

Nuts: almonds, cashews, walnuts, and Brazil nuts, to be exact. Eating 1-2 Brazil nuts per day has been shown to increase serotonin levels.

Fruits and vegetables: It is common knowledge that vegetables and fruits are healthy. The advantages have been frequently stated by parents, in books, and in small pamphlets at the doctor's office. And your mind is not immune to these advantages; eating fresh produce can help lift a low mood. Asparagus, avocado, blueberries, raspberries, and blackberries are particularly effective mood boosters.

Green tea and chamomile: Chamomile tea should be consumed before going to bed because it promotes restful sleep. This means you might be able to sleep without feeling anxious or uncomfortable. Green tea has a long list of health benefits, including aiding in the treatment of depression. Drink at least two cups of green tea per day.

Whole wheat bread The cottage cheese Oatmeal

Brain Food: Consume a lot of omega-3-rich foods, as this essential fatty acid can improve your mood. This fatty acid is particularly abundant in olive oil and most seafood.

Change in diet: cut back on sugar.

When it comes to your mood, diet is just as important as exercise. What you put into your body has a significant impact on your overall mental state.

Inflammation is the leading cause of depression, anxiety, and other mental disorders. Consuming too much gluten and/or sugar causes inflammation. This cause is subtle because we don't usually associate mood disorders with the foods we eat. According to research, the majority of people who suffer from mood disorders are gluten-sensitive. Food is literally intended not only for your body but also for your brain. This is why we must eat a variety of nutritious foods.

Keep your distance!

The foods listed below may contribute to the worsening of depression and the prevention of mood improvement. You should avoid the following foods:

Refined Sugar: Eating sugary foods will make you feel good for a short time as you enjoy the divine sugar rush. This, however, will not last because the inevitable sugar crash will hit you like a ton of bricks. This can make you sluggish and lethargic.

Artificial Sweeteners: Avoid drinks and foods containing artificial sweeteners because they can contribute to a depressive state.

Alcohol: Alcoholic beverages have a depressant effect. This means that an ice-cold glass of beer can actually contribute to a chemical imbalance in your brain. Regular drinking, especially binge drinking, will lower your serotonin levels over time, which is the neurotransmitter responsible for your mood state.

Alcohol will also heighten your anxiety and stress levels. Finally, when it comes to mood, drinking alcohol is a vicious cycle. A person drinks to feel good and relax, but alcohol actually depresses your mood over time. Regardless, people will reach for the bottle in search of that good feeling and a way to get rid of their sadness. That is where the vicious cycle begins. If you are depressed, it is best to avoid alcohol for at least a short period of time.

Caffeine: Studies have shown that people who consume an excessive amount of caffeine are more likely to suffer from depression than those who do not consume caffeinated beverages. With a world full of coffee and tea drinkers, abstaining from caffeine entirely is a tall order. As a result, it is best to consume caffeinated beverages in moderation. Limit your intake to 2-3 cups of coffee or 3–4 cups of tea per day.

Chapter 9
Changes in Lifestyle to Combat Depression

Depression is difficult for anyone. Aside from eating healthy foods and changing your mindset, there are some lifestyle changes you should make to combat depression in 30 days:

1. Exercise

Going to the gym or even going for a 30-minute walk can significantly improve your mood.

Exercise produces hormones that help fight depression. It acts as a natural antidepressant. Duke University conducted a study that revealed that 30 minutes of exercise per day for up to 4 months helped people with depression by improving their mood, reducing stress, providing a good night's sleep, and boosting self-esteem. Physical activity causes brain chemicals to be released that promote relaxation and euphoria. Exercise relieves the tension that contributes to depression. When you exercise, you will also feel a lot better about your appearance, which will boost your confidence.

Put on your running shoes, neon spandex dancing gear, or flashy swimsuit and get moving. Being active for only 20–30 minutes per day can significantly improve your mood. This is because exercise increases serotonin levels while also releasing endorphins. Exercise is a simple and inexpensive way to combat depression. Try to vary it so that monotony does not set in. The last thing you want is for the exercise that is supposed to make you happy to turn into a tedious chore that you dread. So, on a sunny Saturday, hike through beautiful mountain trails, swim laps on Tuesday and go for a run on Thursday. Have some fun with it.

The Advantages of Exercise and the Different Types Available

According to one study, depression and exercise have a link. As individuals

They feel better when they move and produce endorphins; exercise improves their mood and helps them concentrate.

Exercise's Psychological Advantages

Endorphins are released into the body when you exercise. It alleviates the sensation of pain in your body. It also produces a pleasant sensation in your body. It is possibly related to morphine. Many people report feeling "euphoric" or "runner's high" after a quick run. They are much more alive, and this is accompanied by a positive outlook.

Endorphins are known as "natural analgesics" because they reduce the sensation of pain. They are produced in the spinal cord, brain, and other parts of the body where neurotransmitters are present. Endorphins bind to the same neuron receptors that pain medications bind to. The advantage of endorphin is that it is not addictive like morphine.

Regular Exercise Has Many Advantages:

Improve your self-esteem Reduce your stress.

Depression and anxiety are pushed away. lowers blood pressure

improves heart health boosts energy levels Bone building and strengthening

Strength and muscle tone are improved. Body fat is reduced.

makes you fit and healthy.

Exercise is not commonly used as a treatment for mild depression. Certain types of exercise are more beneficial to people suffering from depression:

dancing, biking, gardening, golfing

Aerobics for Housework Walking, swimming, and yoga work in the yard

Joining a group therapy class may be beneficial for people suffering from depression because it provides a much-needed support group. You could also work out with your friends. Doing group exercises will provide you with emotional comfort because you will know that you are not alone.

Joining exercise classes is fine if you've always been active. However, if you are not active, are over 50 years old, or have medical conditions, it is best to consult with your doctor before beginning an exercise program.

Do you want to know how often you should exercise to relieve the symptoms of depression? Endorphins are activated by at least 30 minutes of exercise three times per week. More exercise is better if you have a lot of time. It is best to start slowly if you are just starting out.

Before beginning an exercise program, consider an easy routine that you can maintain and follow. It can be dancing, running, or anything else you enjoy doing as long as you are comfortable with the activity and the time commitment. If you want to get started right away, try to incorporate it into your daily routine. Schedule it and add it to your to-do list for the day. Variety is essential. Make a schedule if you used to play multiple sports when you were younger. Try to mix and match to find people with whom you can work out. When it comes to exercise, do not overspend. Canvass first before purchasing gym memberships. Exercise on a regular basis as well. Exercise must become a habit in order to combat depression.

2. Loss of weight

Losing weight benefits both your overall health and your self-esteem.

It also provides much-needed mental clarity. You are not required to drastically reduce your weight. You can eat well and exercise regularly. There's no need to try a fad diet. It will not benefit you, and the weight you will lose is unlikely to be permanent. When you resume your normal eating habits, it will return with a vengeance. Do not fall for fad diets that require you to consume a specific juice or type of food for a week in order to lose weight. You should eat nutritious foods to help you relax.

3. Sleep

Fatigue from sleep deprivation can exacerbate depression symptoms.

People suffering from depression have difficulty sleeping. Lying awake at night is difficult, especially when your brain refuses to calm down. There may also be times when you wake up for no apparent reason and are unable to return to sleep. Create a bedtime routine that adheres to a sleep schedule in order to get some shut-eye.

Change your sleep routine to get a good night's sleep. Try to get 8–10 hours of sleep per day. Sleep in a very dark room, turn off all electric devices, and wake up without an alarm to improve the quality of your sleep. Waking up without an alarm can be difficult at first, but it is a simple habit to develop. Try to sleep 8–10 hours before you need to wake up; this will help you wake up naturally.

It has been discovered that depression and insomnia are related.

Depression is rooted in the neuro-physical processes of the body and can have a direct impact on sleeping patterns. In fact, one of the primary symptoms of depression is an inability to sleep or a lack of sleep.

People who are depressed describe their experience as arduous, especially when they are unable to sleep at night. Sleep, like food and shelter from natural forces, has been a fundamental aspect of human life for as long as it has been a necessity for many other organisms. Our bodies require recharge and rejuvenation in order to function properly in daily life. Sleep allows our organs, particularly the neurotransmitters in our brains, to rest and replace worn-out cells. However, this does not imply that the entire body is temporarily shut down. It is still operational. Sleep simply limits physical energy, giving worn-out cells more time to rejuvenate.

Going to bed at the reasonable hour of 10:30–11pm may appear tedious, but getting 7-8 hours of sleep per night can have a significant impact on your mood. If you stay up late glued to the internet [Tumbler, I'm looking at you], you will most likely be cranky and irritable, and it will worsen your depression in the long run. Hours of peaceful and calm sleep are critical to your plan to kick depression in the shins. It is obvious that sleep is an essential part of life. Sleep deprivation can have both emotional and biological consequences that are far from insignificant.

Sleep deprivation

Patients suffering from depression find it difficult to sleep at night because their thoughts that cause melancholy keep them awake.

Some people said it's difficult to get them to sleep, while others said it's difficult to stay asleep. Others, on the other hand, experience daytime sleepiness as a result of staying awake at night.

It can be difficult to balance trying to stay productive with having a stable career. People who are depressed are not at their most efficient when they are sleep-deprived. When insomnia has taken over one's consciousness, the depression worsens.

Sufferers also report paranoia as a side effect of their insomnia. Due to a lack of rest and the time required to replace worn-out cells, the mind will react to certain stimuli in unusual ways. Insomniacs will struggle to maintain a logical flow of thought.

As a result, awkward conversations and an inability to socialize with colleagues occur. Some sufferers are easily irritated by the smallest things and may appear rude and misunderstood to others in the workplace.

Sufferers are prone to nausea on a biological level. They may also appear limp and experience discomfort in certain limbs.

Getting some sleep

There is no doubt that sleep is an essential part of daily human life, and it may even be a cure for depression.

It is possible to be depressed while sleeping enough. And, by allowing your mind to relax, sleep may be an effective treatment. Sleep can also make your mind less agitated by the thoughts that keep you awake.

If you are experiencing sleeping difficulties, speak with your doctor, who may prescribe appropriate medication.

Limiting caffeine consumption and eating a well-balanced diet are also important steps in combating sleep deprivation.

4. Relationships

It is best if you reach out to your loved ones and friends for assistance in overcoming this problem.

Individuals can suffer from depression. Supportive people who promote positivity will help you get through difficult times in your life.

5. Read each day.

According to research, reading for just a half hour a day can provide numerous benefits. Reading promotes serenity and relaxation.

Reading spiritual books can lower your blood pressure and relax you. Reading self-help books can help people cope with pain and mood disorders. Reading improves both mental stimulation and brain memory. Reading a book requires mental effort, which allows you to train your brain. To improve, the brain requires exercise (just like a muscle).

Other advantages of reading include stress reduction, increased knowledge and vocabulary, improved concentration, improved writing skills, and improved analytical skills.

6. Try not to isolate yourself.

When you surround yourself with people, you don't give in to all of your negative thoughts.

Speaking with a trusted friend, support group, or family member can lift your spirits and make you feel better about yourself. When you don't feel motivated to deal with your depression, you need a supportive mastermind to lift you up. Also, try to add value whenever you interact with others. Positivity, someone who listens to others, helping others, or even a smile can all provide value. Adding value relieves stress and allows you to focus on other things.

Most people who are depressed make the mistake of cutting themselves off from the outside world. And we don't mean attempting to isolate oneself from a society on which one is completely reliant. However, it entails attempting to avoid any social contact with friends, family members, or people who simply wanted to help you get through the depression.

Depressed people blame the world's decisions for their condition to turn against them, that it is uncontrollable no matter how hard we try. Patients are oblivious to the fact that the world operates in mysterious ways. We are not always able to obtain the desired grade, promotion, or attract our childhood crush. The universe revolves around probabilities, but most of us try to deny this fact.

We might as well rebel against the world, don't you think? But will it actually help?

Conditions, conditions, conditions

People who are depressed believe they are vulnerable, which explains their low self-esteem and lack of motivation to do anything productive. And we can always assume that cultivating social relationships is a fruitful endeavor.

We require people in the same way that plants require sunlight to survive. By denying yourself any social interaction, you are attempting to persuade the world that you do not require friends or family to enjoy your life. Some melancholic patients will even go so far as to claim that their friends and family contributed to their depression, but this is merely an illusion.

Social Requirements

Man has always been a social animal because it is built into his nature. He can benefit from a meaningful relationship with his coworker. Aside from material things, having a friend can make one feel safe.

Depressed people have always failed to recognize that attempting to isolate themselves can help them become better people than when they were surrounded by the warmth of human company. The reality is that this assumption has a negative impact.

Depriving yourself of any contact with your friends and loved ones will only deepen and morph your emotional crisis. Without any emotional refuge to turn to, convincing yourself that only you can end the misery can only lead to an extended period of boredom.

The desire to be alone is not justified by sadness. Depression can be a personal confrontation, but it will take help from others who are close to you and understand your problems to overcome the problem before it begins to overwhelm your impulses.

Spend time with others.

Having fun with your friends and family will help you recover from depression carry out the desired effect

Your mind needs to unwind, and nothing but a healthy conversation with your best friend or a hearty meal with your parents can help you survive the depression.

7. Take Part

Allowing yourself to engage in mental and physical labor can help you gradually reduce the effects of depression.

You must skulk because you are depressed. Sadness depletes a significant amount of energy required for productive and recreational work.

To put it succinctly, depression makes you feel completely useless. You will eventually try to convince yourself that life isn't worth living because it's boring and absurd.

This only leads to a paradox. The longer you stay idle, the more melancholy you become, which gives you a perceived reason to stay idle. Furthermore, your mind will suffer as a result of having no other tasks to complete and being engulfed by depression.

The situation worsens over time until the sufferer declares that enough is enough.

This problem can be solved through action.

Taking Care of Your Career

A person with a job may find it difficult to carry out his or her duties and tasks at work. Sadness tries to bring him down and demotivates him from performing his daily tasks effectively. He is also forced to avoid all contact with his coworkers. The negative impact of this is that his reputation within the workplace suffers, as does his ability to earn more opportunities.

If you truly believe that your job has become lonely and monotonous, you may need to reconsider. Look to your career for a suitable cure that will enable you to get back on your feet and become the life of the office once more.

You can do so by focusing your attention on your daily tasks. When your mind is preoccupied with work, it is easier to focus on other things and begins to set aside thoughts that contributed to the depression.

8. Mental Exercise

In your spare time, try to engage in recreational and intellectual activities.

Work cannot be your sole source of relief from the effects of depression.

Read a book, solve a crossword or sudoku puzzle, or, if you're not alone, strike up an interesting conversation with someone else in the room. Any of these activities can help take your mind off the things that make you sad while also stimulating your cognitive faculties.

9. Hobbies are important.

You should also pursue your favorite hobbies, particularly those that are creative.

You can never go wrong with engaging in your creative passions, whether it's painting, writing songs, or composing poems.

Using these, you can effectively express yourself in a way that suits you.

Creative work also encourages you to free your mind from anything that makes you unhappy. It also appears to be a form of therapy in that it allows you to express your sadness on paper or canvas. This is a tried-and-true method that psychologists recommend to their patients.

10. experiment with new things.

Take the risk of trying new things, and your mind may find a reason to forget about being depressed.

If your depression is so severe, you might as well try a different approach. That is to say, try new things.

Do you want to skydive or bungee jump all the time? Or do you have a strong desire to visit a place you've never visited before?

11. Avoid negative individuals.

Negative people tend to depress you emotionally.

When you are vulnerable to negative thoughts, a negative person can undo all of your hard work to become and stay positive in an instant. When you spend enough time with negative people, no matter how strong your willpower is, your subconscious will latch on and take over mindsets. This will cause you to become extremely negative. So avoiding negative people and gradually removing them from your life is the best way to deal with them. If the negative person is difficult to avoid, there are other techniques for avoiding them subtly. Some methods:

First and foremost, avoid engaging with their negativity.

It's easy to get sucked into someone's negativity. But don't get involved. Not engaging does not imply that you simply ignore that person, but rather that you maintain an emotional distance from them. When someone focuses on negative talk, choose a brief response. You don't have to be rude again. Answering quickly, casually, and positively is the ideal combination!

Be encouraging.

Be willing to listen to the person with a compassionate ear and offer assistance if they request it (don't try to force your beliefs on them; this rarely works)! Sometimes someone simply has a bad day or period and requires assistance. If the person's negativity persists on the same topic, it's time to distance yourself from them.

Positive thinking will disarm their negativity.

The best way to disarm their negativity is to redirect it toward positive topics. Don't be abrupt, as this may give the impression that you don't care about them. Be subtle and gently redirect the conversation with something amusing or a well-intended compliment.

Reduce your alone time between the two of you.

When you're hanging out with the negative person, try to do so in groups. This will allow the negative person to take over the group's positivity. It also makes things easier for you because the person's negativity is directed not only at you but at the entire group.

Establish limits.

Recognize that their negativity is not your fault. If they continue to depress you, it's time to avoid them as much as possible. If it's a coworker, cut them off. If it is a family member, try to spend time away from them or even refuse to answer their phone calls.

www.ingramcontent.com/pod-product-compliance
Lightning Source LLC
Chambersburg PA
CBHW070303220526
45465CB00004B/1730